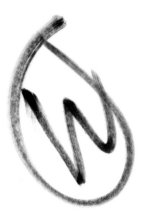

SCIENCE AND SOCIETY™

TECHNOLOGY AND INFERTILITY

ASSISTED REPRODUCTION AND MODERN SOCIETY

Linda Bickerstaff

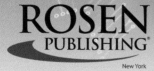

ROSEN
PUBLISHING®

New York

Published in 2009 by The Rosen Publishing Group, Inc.
29 East 21st Street, New York, NY 10010

First Edition

Library of Congress Cataloging-in-Publication Data

Bickerstaff, Linda.
Technology and infertility : assisted reproduction and modern society / Linda Bickerstaff.
  p. cm.—(Science and Society)
Includes bibliographical references and index.
ISBN-13: 978-1-4358-5024-8 (library binding)
1. Human reproductive technology—Juvenile literature. 2. Infertility—Treatment—Juvenile literature. I. Title.
RG133.5.B53 2009
618.1'78—dc22

                                                                    2008013569

Manufactured in Malaysia

On the cover: A technician withdraws deep-frozen cells for in vitro culturing in a laboratory.

CONTENTS

A ccording to the U.S. Census Bureau, the world's population was 6,641,114,623 on January 1, 2008. This number was almost thirty-nine million more than the number on the same date in 2007. About three hundred million of these people live in the United States. There is one live birth every eight seconds in the United States; a person dies every eleven seconds. One person immigrates (legally) to the United States every ten seconds. As a result, there is a net gain in the population of the United States of (at least) 11,585 people every day.

A report from the Centers for Disease Control and Prevention (CDC), released on December 7, 2007, says that in 2006 there were a total of 4,265,996 births in the United States. That was 127,647 (3 percent) more births than were reported in 2005. The same report emphasizes that the teen birth rate rose for the first time since 1991 and was forty-two births per one thousand girls between the ages of fifteen and nineteen. Eighteen- and nineteen-year-old teens had a birth rate of seventy-three births per one thousand girls. The number of teen pregnancies each year is about three times the number of births. One-third of teens elect to have abortions, and about one-third experience spontaneous miscarriages of their pregnancies.

With these statistics in mind, it is hard to imagine that infertility is of particular concern to anyone. It is not a concern to nations that are struggling to feed and house their exploding populations. Teens, faced with unintended pregnancies, are not worried about infertility. It is a major health issue, though, for

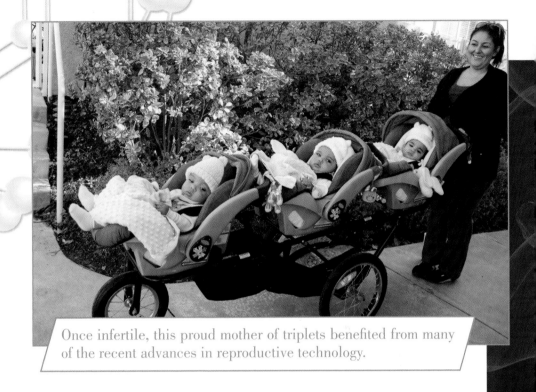

Once infertile, this proud mother of triplets benefited from many of the recent advances in reproductive technology.

as many as one in six couples in the United States who desperately want children and seem unable to have them.

Infertility is defined as the inability to get pregnant within twelve months, despite having frequent and unprotected sexual intercourse. The authors of an article on infertility from the Mayo Clinic say, "Overall, after 12 months of unprotected intercourse, approximately 85 percent of couples will become pregnant. Over the next thirty-six months, about 50 percent of the remaining couples will go on to conceive spontaneously." This still leaves many couples unfulfilled in their desire to have children.

For many years, adoption was the only way that an infertile couple could build a family. Today, there is a new science of procreation. Debora Spar, in her book *The Baby Business*, says, "It [the new science] is a modern phenomenon, a post-industrial miracle that emerged from the high technologies of bio-chemistry, microsurgery, and genetic engineering." With advancements in reproductive technology, infertile couples now have several options for meeting their goals of conceiving and bearing children. They are also faced with more physical, emotional, ethical, and legal issues than ever before. Procreation was once a private and very personal matter between marital partners. It is now a public societal debate dealing with "test tube babies" and "designer kids."

Many controversial side issues have been created by reproductive technology. These include embryo adoption and the use of cryo-preserved (frozen) embryos in stem cell research. Are advancements in reproductive technology changing the way society views procreation? Are children becoming a commodity to be bought and sold? These are a few of the questions being raised for which there are no answers. Yesterday's science fiction is today's reality.

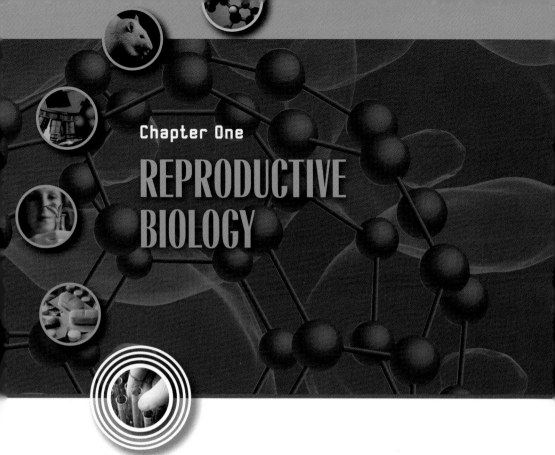

Chapter One
REPRODUCTIVE BIOLOGY

When you stop to consider all the biological functions that must occur at just the right time to create a child, it is amazing that the process works at all—and yet it does. Simplistically, all it takes is a fertile male, a fertile female, and perfect timing.

Female Reproductive Anatomy

The basic components of a woman's reproductive system are two ovaries, two fallopian tubes, and a uterus. The uterus is a muscular organ whose primary function is to house and nurture a developing embryo. The fallopian tubes are narrow conduits, or

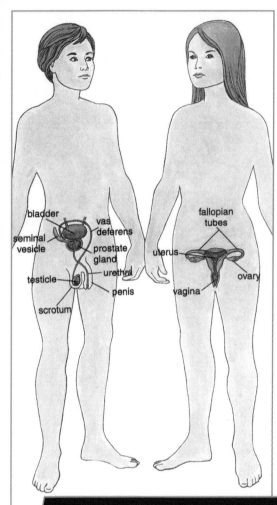

bladder
seminal vesicle
vas deferens
prostate gland
testicle
urethra
penis
scrotum
fallopian tubes
uterus
ovary
vagina

The male and the female reproductive systems, as illustrated here, depend on hormones from other organs in the body to function properly.

channels, that carry eggs from the ovaries into the uterus. The tubes are attached at one end to the top of the uterus. The free ends of the tubes are funnel-shaped and have finger-like projections that surround the ovaries to sweep eggs into the tubes.

A woman's ovaries are walnut-sized organs consisting of thousands of clusters of cells called primordial follicles. In the center of each follicle is a single ovum, or egg—the female gamete. Females are born with all of the ova (about one or two million) that they will ever have. Over the course of a woman's reproductive life, only three hundred to four hundred ova will mature and be shed (ovulated) from the ovaries. The rest simply die and are reabsorbed into the woman's body.

A girl's reproductive life begins at menarche, the time at which she begins to ovulate and have monthly episodes of bleeding called menstruation. Menarche usually occurs at age twelve or thirteen, although it can occur as early as eight or nine years old. By about age fifty, a woman has reabsorbed or used all of her ova and is no longer fertile. She undergoes menopause and stops menstruating. During the intervening years, a woman has menstrual cycles every twenty-five to thirty-six days (the average is twenty-eight days) unless she becomes pregnant. During each menstrual cycle, an egg matures and bursts out of its follicle. It is swept into a fallopian tube and carried toward the uterus, the lining of which has thickened during the cycle. If a sperm fertilizes the egg as it travels along the fallopian tube, the resulting embryo implants in the uterus and begins to grow. If the egg is not fertilized during that cycle, it does not implant. It is lost as the lining of the uterus sloughs off, leading to menstruation.

Male Reproductive Anatomy

Testicles (testes) are the male reproductive organs that produce male gametes (sperm). The testes are suspended in a sac of skin and connective tissue called the scrotum. Each testis connects to a coil of tubules, the epididymis, in which sperm are held until they mature. Each epididymis connects to a long duct called the vas deferens. The vasa (ducts) are attached to the urethra, the tube that lies within the spongy portion of the penis and carries urine out of the body. During sexual intercourse, sperm move out of each epididymis, through the vas deferens, and into the urethra. Along the way, they mix with fluids from several glands to form seminal fluid or semen. Seminal fluid is pushed out of the body during ejaculation.

Boys tend to reach sexual maturity between the ages of thirteen and fifteen. After that, they produce millions of sperm each day. Although sperm production declines with age, most men remain fertile throughout their lifetimes.

Timing Is the Key

Assuming that both partners produce normal gametes, timing becomes the key element in conception. An egg and sperm have to merge at just the right time and in just the right place for normal

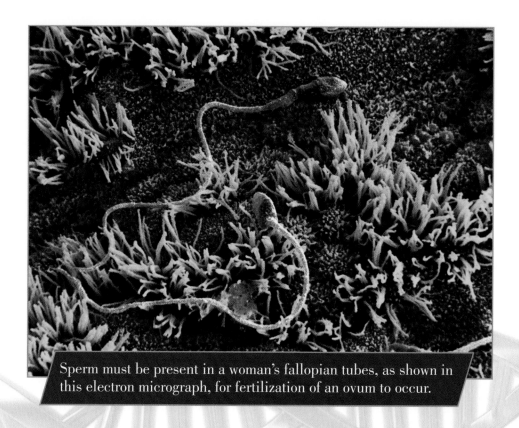

Sperm must be present in a woman's fallopian tubes, as shown in this electron micrograph, for fertilization of an ovum to occur.

conception to occur. The place is a fallopian tube, where the egg is fertilized by a single sperm.

The timing of the process involves the interaction of several hormones. A hormone is a chemical substance produced and secreted by one organ in the body that affects the function of other organs of the body. The four most important hormones in reproduction are follicle stimulating hormone (FSH), luteinizing hormone (LH), estrogen, and progesterone. FSH and LH are secreted by the pituitary gland, a small structure that sits just beneath the brain. Estrogen and progesterone are secreted by ovaries. When these four hormones are secreted in the correct

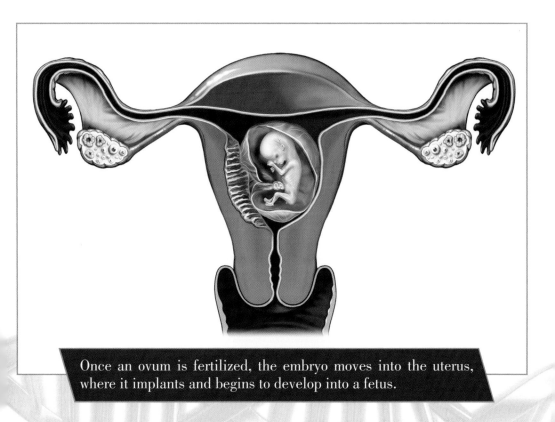

Once an ovum is fertilized, the embryo moves into the uterus, where it implants and begins to develop into a fetus.

amounts and at the right time, a woman will ovulate on about day fourteen of her menstrual cycle. To maximize the possibility of the egg being fertilized, a couple should have intercourse on days thirteen, fourteen, and fifteen of the cycle. Eggs live for only twenty-four hours after ovulation, so the window of opportunity for fertilization is small. Sperm can actually "hang around" within the woman's reproductive tract for forty-eight to seventy-two hours following intercourse. If fertilization occurs, an embryo is formed. The embryo then usually moves into the uterus, where it implants and grows into a fetus.

MYTHS AND FACTS

MYTH It is not difficult to get pregnant.

FACT A healthy couple, in their prime reproductive years, has a 25 percent chance of conceiving with each menstrual cycle. Only 50 percent of couples conceive within six months of starting to have intercourse. Eighty-five percent conceive within one year. The remaining 15 percent of couples have difficulty and may never conceive.

MYTH Childless couples who adopt a child will have a better chance of conceiving a child after the adoption than they did before the adoption.

FACT Studies show that would-be parents who believe they are infertile and adopt a child have a 5 percent pregnancy rate following adoption. This is the same pregnancy rate reported in couples who think they're infertile and did not adopt.

MYTH The timing of intercourse has nothing to do with conception.

FACT At least 20 percent of couples fail to conceive because they do not understand the importance of timing in a menstrual cycle. They fail to have intercourse during the fertile period of the woman's cycle.

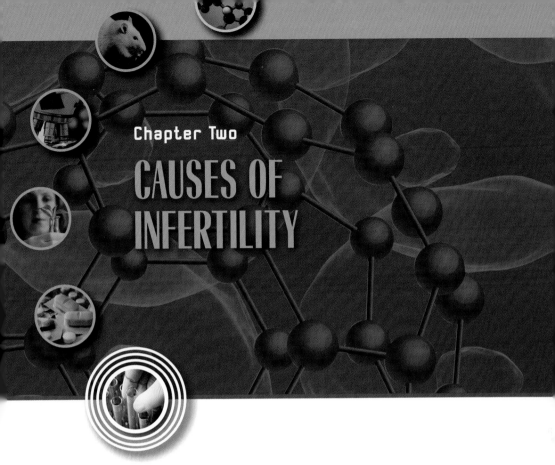

Chapter Two

CAUSES OF INFERTILITY

A llison Van Dusen, in her article "Men's and Women's Fertility Facts—Explained," reports that in 2007 the prevalence of infertility in the United States was as high as one in six couples of childbearing age. Contrary to popular belief, infertility is not exclusively a female problem. Women's health issues account for infertility in about one-third of couples. Another third cannot conceive because of male infertility. A combination of male and female factors accounts for the remaining third of infertile couples. Advanced age, especially that of the female partner, is a key component in the last group. Women have a finite number of ova. When they are gone, they are gone.

Shared Risk Factors for Infertility

The three most important risk factors for infertility in both men and women are advancing age, smoking, and obesity.

Age

Men become less fertile as they age, notes Dr. Harry Fisch, director of the Male Reproductive Center at New York-Presbyterian Hospital/Columbia University Medical Center. Men over thirty-five are twice as likely to be infertile as those under twenty-five. They are also more likely to have children with birth defects due to the decreased genetic quality of their sperm.

Deborah Gaines recounts in the article "Fertility and Your Age" that a woman's fertility peaks between ages twenty and twenty-four. By age thirty-five, her fertility is only 80 percent of what it was at her peak. By age forty-five, a woman may be 95 percent less fertile than she was at age twenty.

Age is particularly significant because couples are marrying at later ages than they did in the past. Couples often wait until they are in their late thirties or early forties before they decide to have children. By then, both women and men are much less fertile than they were in their twenties.

Smoking

Smoking contributes to infertility in women by increasing the rate at which their eggs deteriorate. This leaves fewer ova to mature to ovulation. It also increases a woman's risk for miscarriage and ectopic pregnancy (when the embryo implants inappropriately in the fallopian tube). According to an article published on HealthDay.com, smoking not only affects a woman's fertility, but it may also decrease her daughter's fertility by as much as two-thirds. The chemical by-products of smoking may keep female

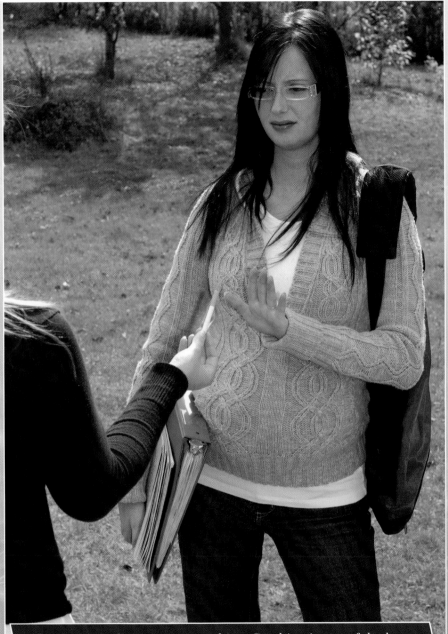

This teen wisely says no to smoking. Smoking is one of the known risk factors for infertility and may also diminish fertility in the daughters of smokers.

fetuses from forming normal amounts of ovarian tissue, so they then have far fewer primordial follicles at birth. Smoking contributes to infertility in men as well. Male smokers have many more misshaped and nonmotile (not capable of moving) sperm than nonsmokers.

Obesity

In the journal *Human Reproduction*, Dr. Jan Willem van der Steeg and his colleagues at the Academic Medical Center in Amsterdam,

How to Calculate Body Mass Index

For metric measurements, calculate as follows:

1. Divide weight in pounds by 2.2 to determine weight in kilograms.
2. Multiply height in inches by 0.0254 to determine height in meters.
3. Multiply height in meters by itself to get meters squared.
4. Divide #1 by #3 to determine body mass index.

For standard measurements, calculate as follows:

1. Multiply weight in pounds by 704.5
2. Divide that product by height in inches squared.

Normal BMI is 18.5 to 24.9 kg/m². A person is overweight if his or her BMI falls between 25 and 30. BMIs of 30 to 40 indicate obesity. Those with BMIs greater than 40 are morbidly obese and are very likely to have major health problems because of their weight.

the Netherlands, published a study on the effects of weight on fertility. The study shows that obese women—those with body mass indices (BMI) greater than 29—were less fertile than women who were not obese. Very obese women—those with BMIs greater than 35—were as much as 43 percent less fertile than normal-weight women. Because 25 percent of women of childbearing age in the United States have BMIs greater than 29, obesity is a major contributing factor to infertility in the country.

William Ledger, professor of obstetrics and gynecology at the University of Sheffield, United Kingdom, as quoted by Dr. van der Steeg, said, "Adult obesity levels have increased four-fold over the last twenty-five years, with two-thirds of adults deemed over-weight." Dr. Ledger believes that the number of couples seeking infertility treatments will double over the next ten years. Obesity will be a major factor contributing to this increase.

Male Infertility

A man may be infertile if he does not produce enough sperm or if many of the sperm he produces are misshaped or nonmotile. If a man's sperm count is lower than ten million sperm per milliliter of semen, he will most likely be infertile. Causes of low sperm production range from serious problems such as pituitary gland dysfunction or genetic disorders to something as simple as spending too much time in the hot tub.

One cause of abnormal sperm production, which should be of particular concern to teens, is the use of anabolic steroids. Anabolic steroids are synthetically made derivatives (products) of the male hormone testosterone. To obtain them legally, a person must have a doctor's prescription. These are the drugs that weight lifters and other athletes use to "bulk up" their muscles and improve their athletic performances. Anabolic steroids are also among the drugs that can cause athletes to be disqualified from athletic events. One side effect of their use, especially in the high doses that are used by athletes and bodybuilders, is infertility.

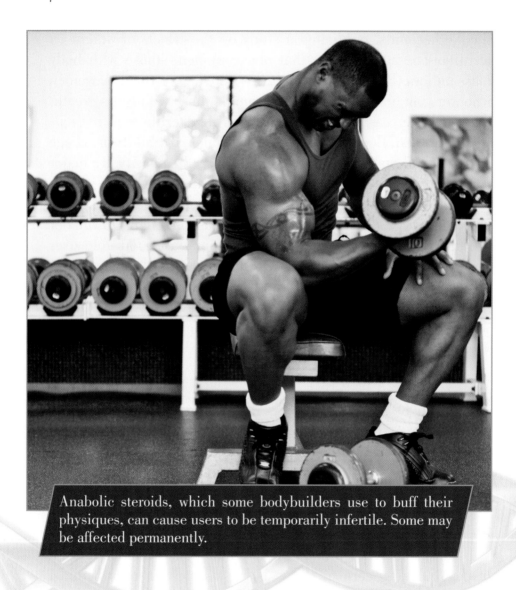

Anabolic steroids, which some bodybuilders use to buff their physiques, can cause users to be temporarily infertile. Some may be affected permanently.

Males who use steroids may notice that their testes get smaller and their breasts enlarge. They stop making sperm, or make only a few that are nonmotile and misshaped. In most men, the process is reversible, with fertility being restored within six to eighteen months after they stop taking steroids. Boys, especially those who use steroids at young ages, may suffer permanent infertility problems.

If a man does produce normal sperm in adequate numbers, he may still contribute to a couple's infertility by not being able to deliver the sperm successfully. Previous infections, especially those caused by sexually transmitted diseases (STDs), can narrow or block the epididymides or vasa deferentia so that no sperm are present in semen. Some men also have trouble obtaining or maintaining erections. Therefore, sexual intercourse is unsuccessful. Male infertility issues occur alone or in combination with female infertility issues in at least 40 percent of couples that are infertile.

Female Infertility

One of the most common causes of infertility in women is the narrowing or blockage of fallopian tubes. Infections, especially with a bacterium called chlamydia, are common causes of this problem. An egg that is fertilized in a damaged tube may not be able to get through the tube into the uterus. The embryo may implant in the tube, leading to a potentially life-threatening tubal (ectopic) pregnancy. If tubes are blocked completely, eggs will

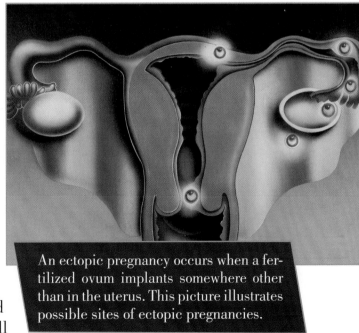

An ectopic pregnancy occurs when a fertilized ovum implants somewhere other than in the uterus. This picture illustrates possible sites of ectopic pregnancies.

never be fertilized. Fallopian tube problems are responsible for 15 to 25 percent of infertility issues in women.

Endometriosis is another cause of female infertility. The endometrium is the lining of the uterus. If some cells of the endometrium move through the fallopian tubes into the abdominal cavity and implant there, a woman has endometriosis. It is a common disorder, occurring in 15 to 25 percent of women between the ages of fifteen and forty-five. Fifty percent of infertile women have the disorder. Endometriosis can contribute to infertility by blocking fallopian tubes and causing hormone imbalances that affect ovulation.

Ovulatory dysfunction, or the failure to produce a mature ovum that bursts from the ovary, occurs in about 40 percent of infertile women. It is usually caused because one or more of the

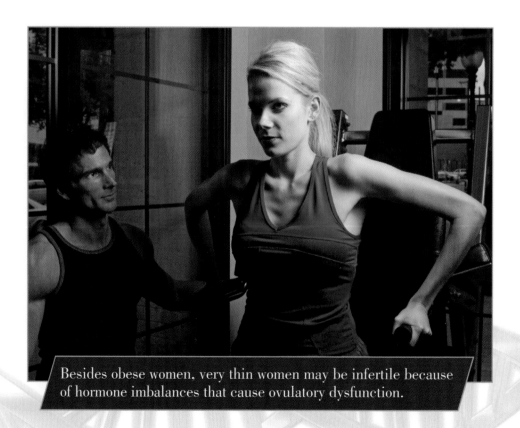

Besides obese women, very thin women may be infertile because of hormone imbalances that cause ovulatory dysfunction.

hormones needed for normal ovulation is out of balance. Obesity is known to cause hormone imbalances and, therefore, contributes to infertility in some women. Women who are very thin or who suffer from the eating disorder anorexia nervosa may also be infertile. Marathon and cross-country runners or ballet dancers, for instance, frequently do not ovulate (or get their periods) because of hormone imbalances. They may be infertile for several years, even after they quit exercising so strenuously and return to a normal weight.

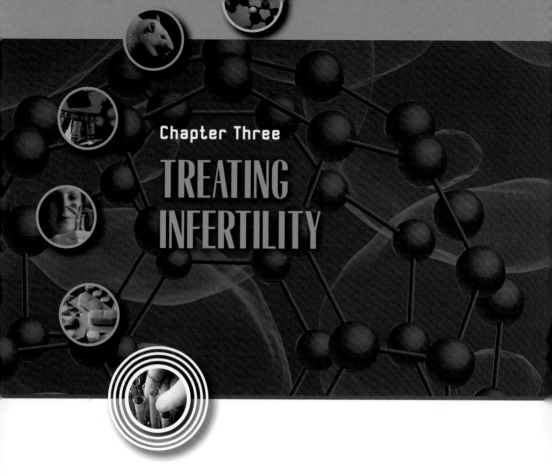

Chapter Three
TREATING INFERTILITY

Daniel Potter and Jennifer Hanin, in their book *What to Do When You Can't Get Pregnant,* say, "Fertility treatments do not make impossible pregnancies possible; they make improbable pregnancies probable." Because each infertile couple has a unique set of problems, a treatment plan must be tailored exclusively for them to maximize the probability of conception.

Define the Problem

The first step in developing a plan to treat infertility is to find its cause(s). The male member of a couple is usually evaluated first, simply because it is less

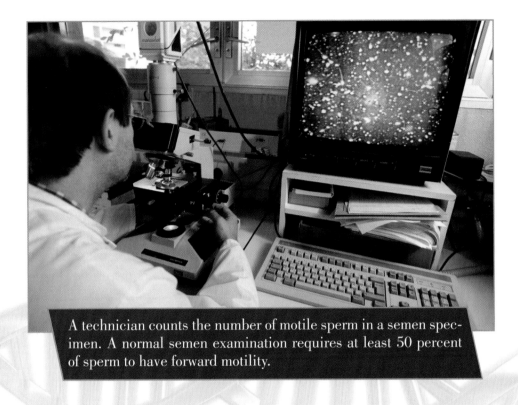

A technician counts the number of motile sperm in a semen specimen. A normal semen examination requires at least 50 percent of sperm to have forward motility.

invasive to do so. A physical examination and a semen analysis, the standards for which are set by the World Health Organization (WHO), are the initial steps. A normal semen specimen must have at least twenty million live sperm in each milliliter of semen. Fifty percent of the sperm must have good forward motility and 30 percent must have normal shapes. If these standards are met, the man should be able to father a child.

A woman's evaluation should occur within a single menstrual cycle. The goal of the evaluation is to obtain three important pieces of information. The first is whether the woman's fallopian tubes are patent (open). The second is whether she ovulates during her menstrual cycle. Assuming she does ovulate, the last piece of information that must be obtained is whether the woman has adequate numbers of follicles remaining in her ovaries to respond to treatment. Proper timing of intercourse should also be evaluated. Once all of these questions have been answered, the couple's doctor can recommend a well-tailored treatment plan.

Treatment Options

Before the development of in vitro fertilization, the first assisted reproduction technique, infertile couples had few options for treatment. The three most effective procedures were intrauterine insemination, ovulation induction, and controlled ovarian hyperstimulation. Many couples still choose to try one or more of these procedures before considering assisted reproduction.

Intrauterine Insemination (IUI)

Intrauterine insemination is a procedure used to maximize the number of healthy sperm that get to the fallopian tubes to fertilize an egg. Sperm deposited into a woman's vagina during sexual intercourse must make a long journey through the uterus and fallopian tubes to reach an egg. Less than 1 percent of the sperm deposited in the vagina reach the uterus alive. Only one-tenth of 1 percent reaches the correct fallopian tube. If concentrated sperm specimens are injected directly into the uterus near the openings to the fallopian tubes, many more sperm are available to fertilize an egg. The procedure is recommended for couples in which the man has a very low sperm count. IUI is thought to increase conception by 7 to 25 percent, depending on the number of normal sperm in the man's semen.

Ovulation Induction

Ovulation induction is initially recommended for infertile women who do not ovulate on a regular basis. Oral medications that stimulate the pituitary gland to secrete large amounts of follicle stimulating hormone (FSH) are prescribed for these women. It is hoped that the high dose of FSH will induce ovulation. Ovulation induction is usually combined with IUI to ensure that large quantities of sperm are available at just the right time to fertilize the egg. Using this combination of treatments, about 8 percent of women get pregnant per cycle of medication. There is a 10 percent increased risk of conceiving twins and less than a 1 percent increased risk of conceiving triplets with ovulation induction.

Controlled Ovarian Hyperstimulation

Not all women with ovulation dysfunction will respond to oral medications. Most, however, will respond to direct stimulation of the ovaries by large doses of injected FSH. If successful, the treatment results in the maturation of three or more follicles at the same time. Women have been known to ovulate as many as twenty to twenty-five eggs during the same cycle with this treatment. When combined with IUI, about 12 percent of women will conceive per cycle.

There are two major risks with ovarian hyperstimulation. The first is the risk of multiple births. The incidence (frequency of occurrence) of conceiving twins increases to 20 percent, and there is a 3 to 5 percent risk of conceiving triplets or more. A woman who carries triplets or more is at significant risk for pregnancy-related medical problems, including high blood pressure, diabetes, blood clots, and blood loss. Extended bed rest or prolonged hospitalization may be required. The babies these women carry are at risk for premature birth and its associated complications.

Professor Emile Papiernik, in the article "Multiple Births: Their Risks and How to Prevent Them," reports that 8 percent of single-birth babies, 42 percent of twins, and 87 percent of triplets are born prematurely (less than thirty-seven weeks' gestation). Deaths around the time of birth are five times more frequent in triplets than in single births. Mental retardation, cerebral palsy,

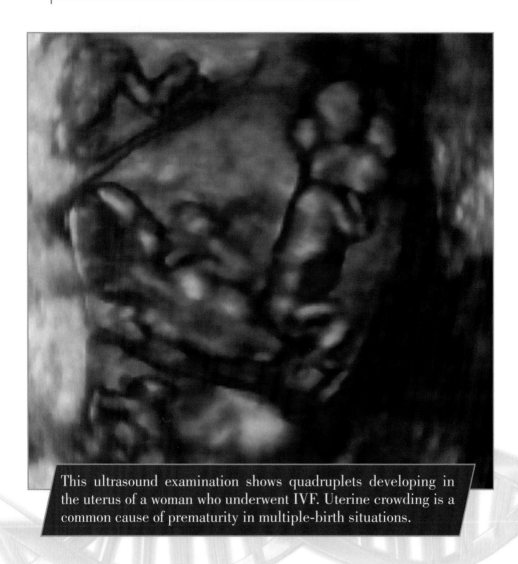

This ultrasound examination shows quadruplets developing in the uterus of a woman who underwent IVF. Uterine crowding is a common cause of prematurity in multiple-birth situations.

and vision and hearing loss are much more frequent in triplets, quadruplets, and quintuplets than in single births.

Before taking medications for controlled ovarian hyperstimulation, a couple should discuss the possible need for multi-fetal reduction with their doctor. Multi-fetal reduction is a procedure that can be done at the end of the first trimester of a pregnancy to reduce the number of fetuses in the uterus. Since overcrowding in the uterus causes many of the problems with multiple births, reducing the number of fetuses to twins makes it more likely that these babies will develop normally. Many couples have difficulty making the decision to have fetal reduction if it has not been considered before conception. They may not accept the procedure because of their religious beliefs. Fetal reduction is forbidden in the Catholic and Islamic faiths and in many Protestant sects. Jewish law sanctions fetal reduction only if a doctor has determined that some fetuses must be eliminated or all will die. Couples who oppose fetal reduction probably should not use controlled ovarian hyperstimulation to treat their infertility unless they are willing to deal with the possibility of multiple births and the inherent risks.

The second major risk in controlled ovarian hyperstimulation is ovarian hyperstimulation syndrome (OHSS). About 33 percent of women getting this treatment experience mild OHSS (nausea and vomiting, and abdominal pain), while 1 percent develops severe symptoms (excess fluid in the abdomen, low blood pressure, and breathing problems). Although rare, deaths have occurred from the syndrome.

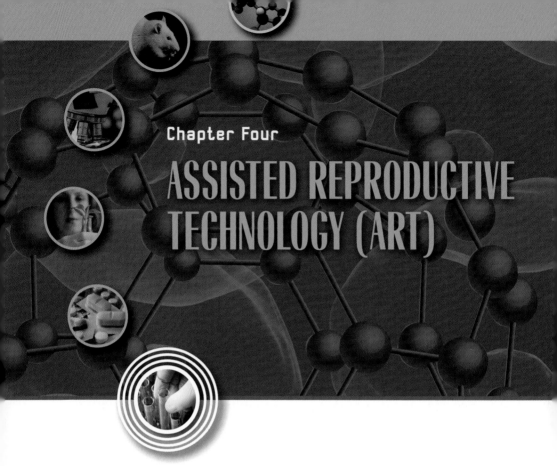

Chapter Four

ASSISTED REPRODUCTIVE TECHNOLOGY (ART)

Assisted reproductive technology (ART) includes any fertility treatment that involves retrieving mature eggs from a woman and fertilizing them with a man's sperm in a culture dish. Selected embryos are then inserted into the woman's uterus, where they will hopefully implant and mature into fetuses. ART should be recommended as the primary choice of treatment for a couple if there is the following:

◇ A female partner over the age of thirty-five.
◇ A female partner with blocked fallopian tubes.
◇ A female partner who does not ovulate.
◇ A male partner who has a low sperm count.

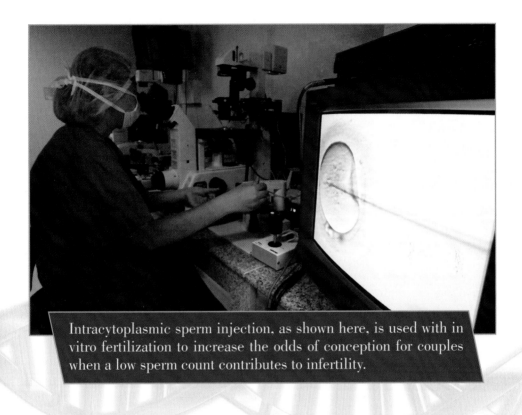

Intracytoplasmic sperm injection, as shown here, is used with in vitro fertilization to increase the odds of conception for couples when a low sperm count contributes to infertility.

Couples who have failed to conceive after three courses of IUI, ovulation induction, and/or ovarian hyperstimulation should also consider ART.

In Vitro Fertilization (IVF)

In vitro fertilization (IVF) started the science of assisted reproductive technology. Robert Edwards, a reproductive endocrinologist, and Patrick Steptoe, a gynecologic surgeon, did the first successful IVF procedure in 1977. Dr. Steptoe harvested a single egg from the ovary of Lesley Brown and placed it in a culture dish. He then placed sperm from her husband, John, into the dish to fertilize the egg. The resulting embryo was transferred into Lesley Brown's

Louise Joy Brown: First Test Tube Baby

Louise Joy Brown, the first child conceived by in vitro fertilization, was born to Lesley and John Brown on July 25, 1978. In spite of the notoriety surrounding her birth, Louise had a happy childhood. Her early education was typical for the child of a middle-class British family. After finishing school, she was a nursery attendant in a child-care center for several years before becoming a postal worker in Oldham, England. Louise married Wesley Mullinder on September 4, 2004, and became a mother at age twenty-eight. Her son, Cameron, who was conceived naturally, was born on December 20, 2006. "He's tiny, just under six pounds [2.7 kg], but he's perfect," the proud mother told the *Mail* (a British newspaper) in a story published on December 24, 2006.

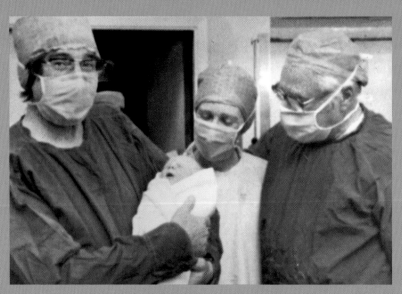

Louise Joy Brown, the first "test tube baby," is held by Dr. Robert Edwards shortly after her birth on July 25, 1978. Dr. Patrick Steptoe is pictured on the right.

uterus, where it implanted and grew. The result was their daughter, Louise Joy Brown. Since 1978, IVF has led to the birth of approximately three million infants worldwide.

The technique of IVF that is used today is very similar to that used by Drs. Edwards and Steptoe. The major difference is that multiple ova, instead of one, are retrieved after a woman undergoes ovarian hyperstimulation. After the eggs are obtained, they are combined with sperm in a laboratory culture dish and placed in an incubator. Three to five days later, the successful embryos are examined under the microscope. Several are selected to be transferred to the woman's uterus. The remaining embryos are frozen for possible future use. About 10 percent of women over the age of forty conceive a child (or children) after an IVF cycle. The procedure is more successful in younger women. About 38 percent of those under the age of thirty-five have babies after an IVF cycle.

It is unusual for all transferred embryos to survive, but they can. This leads to the development of twins or more, depending on the number of embryos transferred. Laura Tarkan, in an article titled "Lowering Odds of Multiple Births," reports that in 1996, 60 percent of IVF cycles included the transfer of four or more embryos to the prospective mother. In 2004, four or more embryos were transferred in only 21 percent of cycles. The reduction in the number of embryos transferred reflects a new appreciation of the risks to both mothers and babies in multi-birth situations and the higher success rates of IVF cycles. The American Society for Reproductive Medicine now recommends that women younger than thirty-five (44 percent of IVF cycles) have one or two embryos transferred, while women older than thirty-seven still have three to five embryos transferred.

Intracytoplasmic Sperm Injection (ICSI)

Intracytoplasmic sperm injection (ICSI) is most often used, in conjunction with IVF, for couples in which the male has a very low

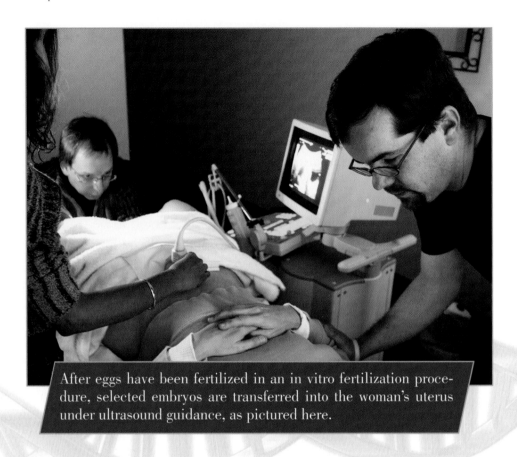

After eggs have been fertilized in an in vitro fertilization procedure, selected embryos are transferred into the woman's uterus under ultrasound guidance, as pictured here.

sperm count. The American Society for Reproductive Medicine's "Patient's Fact Sheet: Intracytoplasmic Sperm Injection (ICSI)," states, "ICSI, a form of micromanipulation, involves the injection of a single sperm directly into the cytoplasm of a mature egg (oocyte) using a glass needle (pipette). This process increases the likelihood of fertilization when there are abnormalities in the number, quality, or function of the sperm." Good motility indicates that sperm are healthy. The best results with ICSI are obtained if very motile sperm are chosen for the procedure. The rate of live births following IVF with ICSI is about 37 percent per IVF cycle, but it may be higher in younger women.

Religious and Ethical Considerations

The Catholic Church has consistently opposed IVF. It believes that reproduction, which is the prime reason for marriage, should be linked to sexual intimacy within a marriage. The Catholic Church also believes that the death of an embryo, which can occur with IVF, is morally the equivalent of killing a person who has already been born. Islamic and Jewish laws, on the other hand, find IVF to be acceptable and desirable for infertile couples. Procreation is very important in these religions, so selected procedures that enable an infertile couple to have children are sanctioned. The egg and sperm used in IVF must, however, come from marriage partners. Hindu and Buddhist authorities also sanction IVF in married couples. IVF is acceptable in most Protestant Christian sects.

IVF has raised several ethical issues. Most involve fertility clinics and how they advertise their results. There is little, if any, oversight of fertility clinics and no standardization in the reporting of results. Some clinics advertise that their procedures are successful if an egg is fertilized and begins to divide, even if it does not result in a successful pregnancy. Other clinics use a live birth as their definition of success. Many people, desperate to have a child, fail to consider a clinic's definition of success and automatically go to the one that advertises the highest success rates. Ethics committees of the various societies dealing with ART are calling for standardization and validation of the reporting of results within the industry.

A Teen Talks About IVF

Sooner or later, all children ask their parents, "Where did I come from?" Couples who undergo IVF to conceive their child must decide if the child needs to be told how he or she was conceived. If they do disclose the information, will the child feel that he or she is different from his or her friends? Or, will that child really care? Tyler Madsen, an IVF-conceived baby, is a spokesperson for the American Fertility Association. In an April 2003 press release from that association, fifteen-year-old Tyler said, "Some people may think that my conception makes me different or special from others. In fact, I'm like any other teenager with the same concerns, the same goals, and the same dreams. I think all kids are special and unique. It doesn't matter how they are conceived. That's just a technicality."

Anne Bernstein, a clinical psychologist and a research associate at the Council on Contemporary Families, agrees with Tyler. In an interview with Jacqueline Stenson for MSNBC, she said, "If both of the adults are the genetic parents of the child, I really don't see disclosure as an issue at all. I don't think it makes any real difference in their [the children's] lives if medical assistance was necessary for fertility."

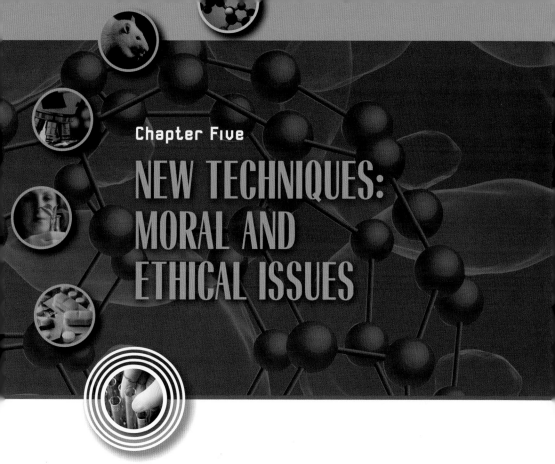

NEW TECHNIQUES: MORAL AND ETHICAL ISSUES

T here are few laws regulating reproductive technology in the United States. There are, however, many moral and ethical concerns about ART. Preimplantation genetic diagnosis (PGD) and microsorting, two techniques that allow the sex of a child to be selected, are among the issues most hotly debated today.

Preimplantation Genetic Diagnosis

Reproductive endocrinologists developed preimplantation genetic diagnosis (PGD) in England in the

35

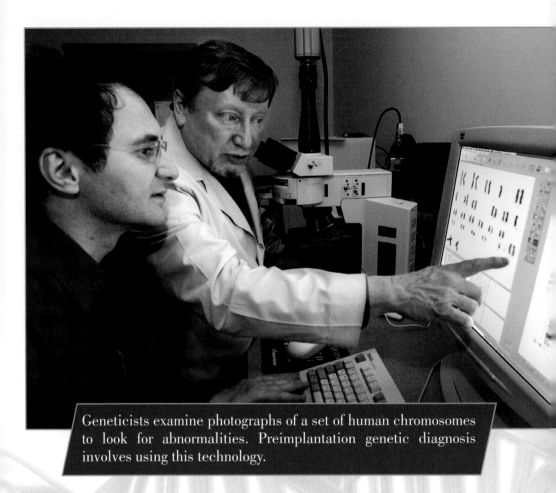

Geneticists examine photographs of a set of human chromosomes to look for abnormalities. Preimplantation genetic diagnosis involves using this technology.

mid-1980s. It was initially developed to identify genetic defects in embryos of women undergoing IVF. The procedure involves removing a single cell from a six-to-eight-cell-stage embryo. The cell is evaluated in a genetics laboratory. Embryos are not damaged by this procedure and make new cells to replace the one removed. Evaluation of the cell can determine if the embryo from which it came has evidence of genetic abnormalities. If it does, the embryo is discarded. If it is normal, it can be transferred to the egg donor's uterus.

Examples of disorders that can occur because of genetic defects include hemophilia, thalassemia, muscular dystrophy, cystic fibrosis, and Down's syndrome, to name a few. Down's syndrome, which is associated with varying levels of retardation, is common in children born to older women, as are most other genetic defects. Some people elect to test their fetuses (whether conceived naturally or via ART) for genetic disorders that run in their families.

Infertile couples that use PGD have fewer children with genetic disorders than do those who do not use PGD. Nevertheless, many people believe that the use of PGD is morally wrong. They believe that life begins when a sperm fertilizes an egg and that discarding genetically defective embryos is a type of murder. Others object to PGD because it allows for gender selection (the ability to choose the sex of an infant). PGD is the single most accurate way of ensuring the sex of a fetus. Many fertility clinics give a couple, in which PGD is being used to check for genetic disorders, the choice of choosing the sex that their baby will be if they conceive. If a couple wishes to have a boy, only embryos with both an X and a Y chromosome will be transferred for implantation. Those wanting girls will get embryos with two X chromosomes.

Microsorting

Microsorting was originally developed to help couples avoid passing sex-linked genetic disorders to their children. A sex-linked genetic disorder is one caused by defective genes attached to either the X chromosome or the Y chromosome. Hemophilia, for instance, is a sex-linked blood disorder that mainly affects males and is caused by genetic abnormalities on the X chromosome.

Today, microsorting is used primarily for family balancing (ensuring that a couple has both male and female children in their family). All female gametes (eggs) have a single X chromosome. One-half of the sperm in a semen specimen will have an X

Indications for Preimplantation Genetic Diagnosis (PGD)

Couples with one or more of the following factors or symptoms should consider preimplantation genetic diagnosis:

- Women older than thirty-five years of age.
- Women with recurrent pregnancy losses.
- Couples with repeated IVF failures.
- Couples in which the male partner has severe male infertility factors requiring ICSI.
- Couples with at least one partner with a family history of an inherited genetic disorder or who is a carrier or is afflicted with a genetic disorder.

chromosome, and one half will have a Y chromosome. If a sperm containing an X chromosome fertilizes the egg, the embryo will have two X chromosomes and will result in a female child. If a sperm containing a Y chromosome fertilizes the egg, the embryo will have one X chromosome and one Y chromosome and will produce a boy.

While working with four species of animals, Dr. Lawrence Johnson, an employee of the U.S. Department of Agriculture (USDA), developed a technique for sorting sperm. Using a technique called flow cytometry, he found that sperm containing the X chromosome could be separated from sperm containing Y chromosomes. When he used sperm specimens that were rich in X chromosome–containing sperm, he greatly increased the number of female offspring born to his animals. By using Y chromosome–enriched sperm samples, he increased the yield of male offspring in his animals.

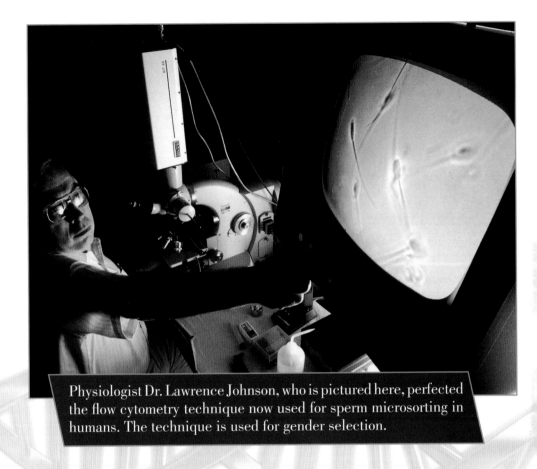

Physiologist Dr. Lawrence Johnson, who is pictured here, perfected the flow cytometry technique now used for sperm microsorting in humans. The technique is used for gender selection.

Scientists at the Genetics and IVF Institute in Fairfax, Virginia, working under Dr. Johnson's guidance, developed a similar technique that could be used in humans. To check to see how accurate the technique would be in producing offspring of a selected gender in humans and to ensure that the procedure was safe to use, a Food and Drug Administration (FDA) clinical trial was begun in 1995. The trial is still ongoing. Recent results show that 92 percent of couples requesting "X-sorts" to increase the probability of conceiving a girl have delivered female babies. "Y-sorts" to increase the probability of having a male child have been successful in 81 percent of couples.

The ethics committee of the American Society for Reproductive Medicine believes that the nonmedical use of preconception gender selection (by microsorting or PGD) should be reserved for families who already have at least one child and want to have a child of the opposite sex for family balancing. This issue is still quite controversial.

Designer Babies: What Teens Think

When PGD and microsorting are used for the purpose of identifying embryos containing abnormal genes or chromosomes, or for choosing the sex of the child to prevent the transmission of sex-linked disorders, most people sanction the use of the techniques. Many, however, disagree with the use of these techniques for nonmedical reasons such as family balancing. In their minds, allowing gender selection is the first step toward allowing couples to "design" their babies.

Do teens have an opinion on designer babies? Anita Shaw and colleagues from the School of Care Sciences, University of Glamorgan, Pontypridd, Wales, believe that young people will have increasing opportunities to use new reproductive technologies to design their babies. Their opinions, however, are rarely sought by agencies developing public policies that may affect those procedures. In 2004, the university established a citizen's jury comprised of fourteen teens. Members of the jury were between the ages of sixteen and nineteen. The jury was asked to consider the following question: designer babies, what choices should we be able to make?

After hearing testimony from thirteen people and seeing a film clip prepared by the British Broadcasting Corporation (BBC), the jury deliberated and reached a "verdict." The jury was in favor of allowing couples to use PGD or microsorting to prevent genetic disorders from being transmitted. The jury members also thought that producing designer babies who could be "savior siblings" (for

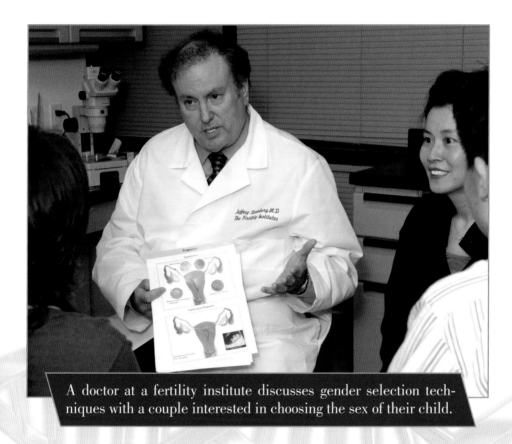

A doctor at a fertility institute discusses gender selection techniques with a couple interested in choosing the sex of their child.

bone marrow transplants, for example) for critically ill brothers or sisters was acceptable. However, this group condemned using ART for gender selection for nonmedical reasons. Jury members subsequently presented their opinions to the Welsh Assembly Government, the Human Genetics Commission, and the Human Fertilization and Embryology Authority of the United Kingdom. Whether the opinions of the jury will affect the regulation of gender selection in the United Kingdom is unknown.

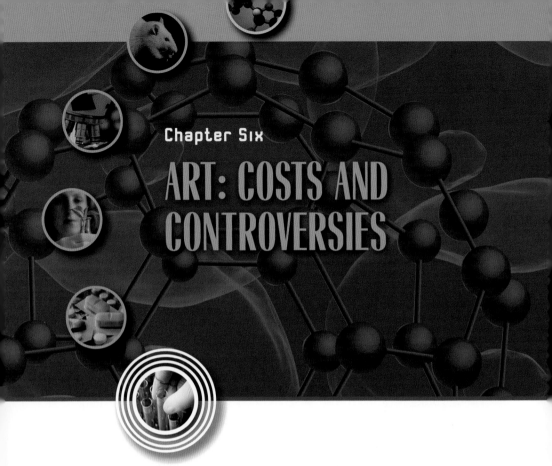

Chapter Six

ART: COSTS AND CONTROVERSIES

F or a fertile couple, the monetary costs of intentionally conceiving a baby are minimal—at the most, the price of a romantic dinner at a favorite restaurant or a weekend getaway. Emotionally, it is a very positive experience. Infertile couples, however, are not so lucky. Conceiving a child with ART is very expensive. It is also an emotional roller coaster and carries no guarantees for success. At the worst, it can sabotage a marriage. A couple may end up not only childless, but also divorced. As an offshoot of helping infertile couples have babies, ART has created unforeseen problems that have become controversial social issues.

The Costs of Creating a Child

In March 2004, the President's Council on Bioethics released a report titled "Reproduction and Responsibility: The Regulation of New Biotechnologies." The report states, "Assisted reproduction is a growing economic enterprise with gross revenues of $4 billion per year, serving one in six infertile couples in the United States." The authors gave these examples of costs for particular procedures:

- **Initial consultation:** $350
- **One IVF cycle using a fresh embryo:** $9,345
- **One IVF cycle using a thawed embryo:** $4,000
- **PGD:** $4,000
- **ICSI:** $2,000

On average, couples try three IVF cycles before they either conceive or give up on the technique. Using the data above, the minimum cost of having a baby using three cycles of IVF (one using fresh embryos and two using frozen embryos, without PGD and ICSI) would be $17,695.

These high costs have created one of the major controversies of assisted reproductive technology: it is not available to everyone who could benefit from it. Most insurance plans do not cover ART, in spite of the fact that infertility is a medical problem. In fourteen states, legislation has required insurance companies to offer coverage for ART, but few policies include all of its costs. Most couples pay for ART out-of-pocket. Those who cannot afford the expense remain childless or consider options such as adoption (which can also be very expensive) or foster parenting.

Third-Party Reproduction

Third-party reproduction refers to reproductive procedures using sperm donation, egg donation, and/or surrogacy. Donated sperm

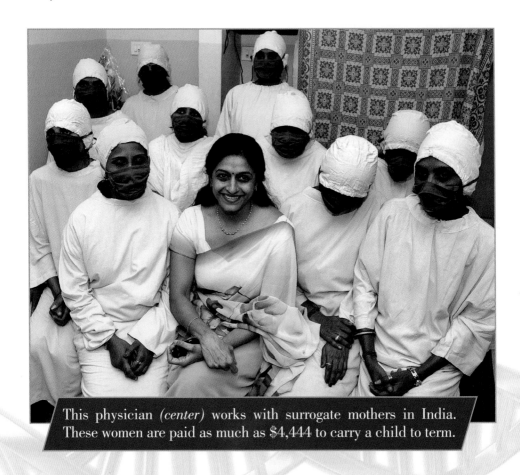

This physician *(center)* works with surrogate mothers in India. These women are paid as much as $4,444 to carry a child to term.

may be used by a couple that is unable to conceive because of male infertility issues. The donated sperm are used to fertilize the woman's egg(s) by intrauterine insemination or by IVF.

Egg donation requires a female donor to undergo ovarian hyperstimulation. After donor eggs are retrieved and fertilized by sperm from the husband of the couple, resulting embryos are transferred to the wife of the couple. Egg donation is most frequently used by couples in which the woman has depleted her supply of eggs and no longer ovulates. It is also used in older couples who have had repeated miscarriages thought to be due to genetically defective eggs.

A traditional surrogate is a woman who donates her own egg(s) to the contracting couple. The egg is fertilized by IUI with sperm donated by the husband of the contracting couple. The surrogate carries the child to birth and then turns the child over to the couple to rear. Gestational surrogacy occurs when the surrogate, or carrier, has no genetic connection to the fetus that she carries. An embryo, derived in one of the four ways, is transferred to her uterus. The four ways in which the embryo may be derived are: 1) from the egg and sperm of the contracting couple; 2) from the wife's egg and donor sperm; 3) from a donor egg and the husband's sperm; or 4) from a donor egg and donor sperm.

Third-party reproduction, and especially surrogacy, is the most controversial issue in ART. Because both sperm and egg donors are paid, and surrogates may receive a considerable amount of money, many feel that third-party reproduction smacks of "baby buying." The Catholic Church and Islamic law forbid it because procreation is reserved for married couples alone. Jewish law is not as clear on this issue, but third-party reproduction is discouraged, especially among Orthodox Jews. Protestant beliefs vary from denomination to denomination.

Third-party reproduction can also be a legal nightmare. Couples who are considering it must know the laws of their state and seek legal help before contracting with a donor or surrogate. If they don't, they may find that the baby they thought was their child is legally the child of another.

Teens Speak About Surrogacy

How do teens born to surrogates feel? Lisa Johnson was conceived using artificial insemination of her father's sperm into a surrogate, who supplied the egg and uterus to carry her. She was thirteen years old in 2003 when her comments were printed in a press release from the American Fertility Association. She said, "I was born through surrogacy and I think it is excellent because couples can have children even if they can't, biologically. It doesn't matter how children are created, as long as they ARE created."

Brian, a fifteen-year-old who has his own blog dealing with surrogacy, feels differently. He says, "My name is Brian, I am the son of a traditional surrogate, a biological father, and an adoptive mother . . . I don't care why my parents and my mother did this. It looks to me like I was bought and sold . . . When you exchange something for money it is called a commodity. Babies are not commodities. Babies are human beings. How do you think it makes us feel to know that there was money exchanged for us?"

Surplus Embryos

Bob Smietana, in an article titled "400K and Counting," reports on a survey of 430 fertility clinics conducted in 2002 by the Society for Reproductive Technology and the RAND Corporation. The survey reveals that there were about four hundred thousand cryo-preserved human embryos, left over from IVF procedures, stored in embryo banks across the country. Eighty-eight percent of these were being stored for future use by the couple that produced them. Nine thousand were waiting to be adopted by other nonfertile couples. Eleven thousand were set aside for scientific research, and the rest were to be thawed and discarded.

The disposition of unused embryos not only raises moral and ethical dilemmas for the couples who create them but also for society as a whole. To keep embryos for possible future use is not initially a controversial issue. It only becomes one when embryos have been frozen for several years and their viability or quality for transfer comes into question. How long an embryo can be frozen and still be safe to use in IVF is not known. Some fertility clinics set a time limit on how long a couple can keep their embryos frozen. If they do not use them or make other plans for them by the end of that time, the fertility clinic allows the embryos to thaw and disposes of them.

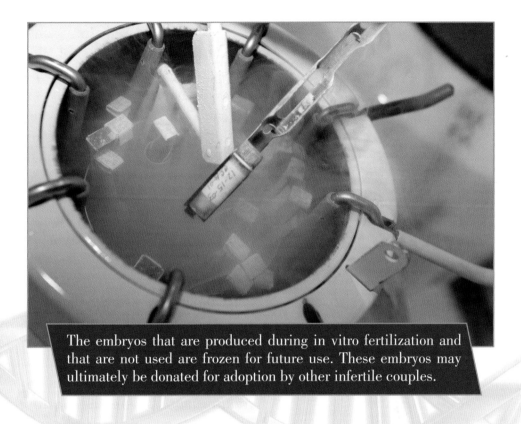

The embryos that are produced during in vitro fertilization and that are not used are frozen for future use. These embryos may ultimately be donated for adoption by other infertile couples.

The Catholic Church does not speak directly about the issue of discarding embryos because it considers ART, and all of its ramifications, to be unacceptable. The destruction of extra embryos is permissible by Jewish law if it is done passively by letting them thaw and die on their own. In most Protestant faiths, disposition of embryos is a personal concern of the couple involved.

Embryo Adoption

Many couples are choosing to put their unused embryos up for adoption. Several agencies across the United States arrange for frozen embryos to be given to other infertile couples. The adopted

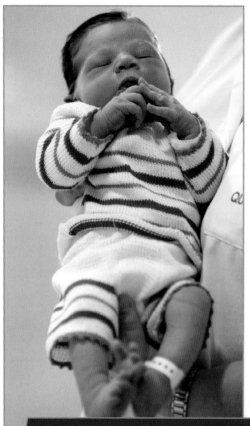

The embryo that eventually became this baby boy was frozen for seven years before the embryo was adopted by a couple (non-biological parents).

embryos are thawed and transferred into the uterus of the "adoptive mother." This procedure eliminates the necessity for ovarian hyperstimulation of the adoptive mother and is cheaper than both IVF and traditional adoption. Costs can run from just under five thousand dollars to around ten thousand dollars.

While embryo adoption is acceptable to many couples who have decided not to use their stored embryos, especially those of Protestant faiths, it is totally unacceptable for Jews and followers of Islamic law. Islamic law does not accept embryo adoption because procreation is only sanctioned between a man and a woman who are married. Because the man who donated the sperm is not married to the woman who will be the child's mother, embryo adoption is not permissible. The objection to embryo adoption, under Jewish law, is that the "adopted" child may unknowingly marry his or her genetic sibling, resulting in incest.

Embryos for Stem Cell Research

The use of frozen embryos in stem cell research has also created much controversy. Until an embryo reaches the sixty-four-cell stage, cells of the embryo are capable of transforming themselves into any of the 220 types of cells in the human body. Researchers are searching for ways to trigger stem cells to develop into specific types of cells. When specific triggers for each type of cell are found, it is hoped that new tissues can be grown to treat persons with diabetes, Parkinson's disease, Alzheimer's disease, and other conditions. This is the ultimate goal of most scientists doing stem cell research today.

Many people believe that this is a laudable goal. Others disagree. When stem cell lines are created from frozen embryos, the embryos themselves are destroyed. For those who believe that life starts when an egg is fertilized, destroying embryos is a type of murder. For these people, the use of frozen embryos for stem cell research is unacceptable. In 2001, U.S. president

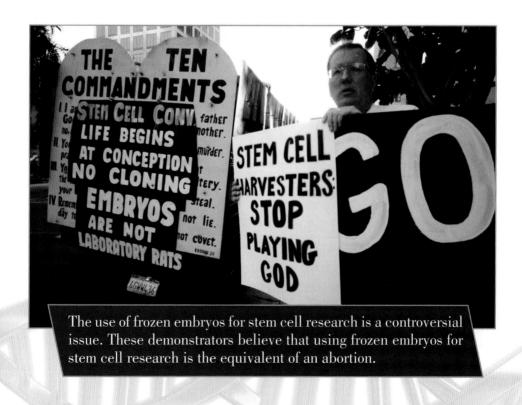

The use of frozen embryos for stem cell research is a controversial issue. These demonstrators believe that using frozen embryos for stem cell research is the equivalent of an abortion.

George W. Bush, who is among those that believe life starts with conception, placed a moratorium on federal funding for stem cell research in which new cell lines were developed from frozen embryos.

The Catholic Church, as well as Jewish law, does not sanction the use of frozen embryos for stem cell research because embryos are destroyed in the process. On the other hand, Islamic law allows the use of frozen embryos for stem cell research that is intended for therapeutic uses as long as prior consent of the couple who created the embryos is obtained.

Summary

Assisted reproductive technology is a four-billion-dollar business that serves one in six infertile couples in the United States. Thirty-seven percent of women under the age of thirty-seven who undergo IVF have a child (or children), whereas only 10 percent of those over the age of forty conceive and bear a child after IVF. Monetary and emotional costs for couples undergoing ART are high, and there are no guarantees of success. There is a high incidence of multiple births with ART. Multiple births increase health risks for both mothers and children. Religious, moral, and ethical concerns are many and varied. There are virtually no federal laws and few state laws regulating ART and little, if any, oversight of fertility clinics. ART now enables parents to choose not only the gender of their child but also the potential physical, mental, athletic, and artistic attributes. Designer children are no longer science fiction; they are a reality. ART is an evolving technology. Where it will lead in the future is anyone's guess. For now, in spite of its many shortcomings, it gives infertile couples hope.

GLOSSARY

anorexia nervosa An eating disorder in which a person has an intense fear of getting fat, refuses to eat, and keeps losing weight. Anorexia nervosa may lead to infertility.

body mass index (BMI) A means of estimating both under-nutrition and over-nutrition. BMI is derived by dividing a person's weight in kilograms by his or her height in meters squared (normal values, 18.9 to 24.5 kg/m).

clinical trials Studies to evaluate the success and safety of medicines, medical devices, or new methods of surgery by monitoring the effects on a large group of people.

conception The moment at which an ovum is fertilized by a sperm to form an embryo.

cystic fibrosis The most common life-shortening inherited disease in the Caucasian population. Boys with cystic fibrosis may be infertile due to congenital absence of the vas deferens.

ejaculation A sudden act of expulsion, as of semen.

endometriosis A condition in which a woman's tissue from the uterine lining (endometrium) grows outside the uterus. When the superficial part of this tissue is shed during menstruation, blood and tissue collect in the abdominal cavity. Endometriosis can cause infertility.

ethical Right and proper; moral; conforming to a professional standard of conduct.

fertilization The act of a sperm penetrating an ovum to form an embryo.

fetus The developing young in the human uterus two months after conception (before eight weeks, it is called an embryo; at birth, it is an infant).

gamete One of two cells, male and female, whose union is necessary in sexual reproduction to initiate the production of a new individual.

hemophilia A hereditary (sex-linked) disorder in which a person's blood will not clot normally.

insemination Introduction of sperm into the female reproductive tract.

invasive Relating to a medical procedure in which the body is entered by puncture or incision.

micromanipulation To examine and skillfully alter a very small object, such as a cell, under magnification with a microscope.

microsorting In family balancing, sperm are sorted under a microscope to separate sperm bearing a female chromosome from those bearing a male chromosome. Insemination using the separated sperm raises the chances of having a child of the preferred gender.

muscular dystrophies A group of inherited disorders characterized by progressive weakening of muscles, frequently leading to death at a young age.

ovum A female gamete; also called an egg.

primordial Earliest or original structure from which an organism is derived; an ovum, for instance.

probable Likely to be or become true or real.

procreation The entire process of bringing a new individual into the world.

sickle cell disease An inherited, life-shortening disease found frequently in people of African descent. Many of the red blood cells (which carry oxygen in the blood) of those with the disease are shaped like sickles, rather than being round. The cells tend to break easily, leading to anemia and other problems.

thalassemia A complex series of inherited disorders that involve underproduction of hemoglobin, the molecules in red blood cells that carry oxygen.

trimester A three-month cycle. Pregnancy is divided into three trimesters.

ultrasound A diagnostic technique in which sound waves are used to visualize internal organs or developing fetuses.

urologist A doctor who specializes in the treatment of the urinary tract.

vagina The canal-like structure extending from the uterus to the outside of the body.

vein A blood vessel that carries blood back toward the heart.

womb Another name for the uterus.

zone pellucida The mucous layer that surrounds an egg that must be penetrated by a sperm before it can fertilize the egg.

zygote An egg after it has been fertilized but before it begins to divide.

American Fertility Association
305 Madison Avenue, Suite 449
New York, NY 10165
(888) 917-3777
Web site: http://www.theafa.org
This association supplies information on reproductive health
   issues affecting infertility.

American Society for Reproductive Medicine
1209 Montgomery Highway
Birmingham, AL 35216-2809
(205) 978-5000
Web site: http://www.asrm.org
This organization is dedicated to helping locate reproductive
   specialists, clinics, and other resources.

Centers for Disease Control and Prevention (CDC)
Reproductive Health Information Source
Division of Reproductive Health
National Center for Chronic Disease and Prevention and Health
   Promotion
4770 Buford Highway, NE, Mail Stop K-20
Atlanta, GA 30341-3717
(770) 488-5200
Web site: http://www.cdc.gov/nccdphp/dhr/index.htm
This is a U.S. government source for information and statistics
   on fertility issues.

Infertility Awareness Association of Canada
2100 Marlowe Avenue, Suite 350

Montreal, QC H4A 3L5
Canada
(514) 484-2891
Web site: http://www.iacc.ca
This patient advocacy group has a nationwide network of support
   groups mandated to promote reproductive health.

Infertility Network
160 Pickering Street
Toronto, ON M4E 3J7
Canada
(416) 691-3611
Web site: http://www.infertilitynetwork.org
This organization provides information, support, and referrals on
   issues related to infertility, miscarriage, and gamete donors.

International Council on Infertility Information Dissemination
P.O. Box 6836
Arlington, VA 22206
(703) 379-9178
Web site: http://www.inciid.org
This organization provides information about the diagnosis,
   treatment, and prevention of infertility.

National Embryo Donation Center
901 Commerce Street
Nashville, TN 37203
(615) 244-2355
Web site: http://www.embryodonation.org
This organization is dedicated to embryo donation and adoption.

Resolve: The National Infertility Association
1310 Broadway
Somerville, MA 02144
(888) 623-0744

Web site: http://www.resolve.org
This national nonprofit organization provides timely support and
information to those suffering from the disease of infertility.

Snowflakes Embryo Adoption Program
801 Chapman Avenue, Suite 106
Fullerton, CA 92831
(714) 278-1020
Web site: http://www.snowflakes.org
This organization deals with issues associated with embryo
adoption.

Society for Assisted Reproductive Technology
1209 Montgomery Highway
Birmingham, AL 35216
(205) 978-5000, ext. 109
Web site: http://www.sart.org
This organization supplies information on the treatment of infertility problems.

Web Sites

Due to the changing nature of Internet links, Rosen Publishing
has developed an online list of Web sites related to the subject
of this book. This site is updated regularly. Please use this link
to access the list:

http://www.rosenlinks.com/sas/tein

FOR FURTHER READING

Farmer, Nancy. *The House of the Scorpion*. New York, NY: Simon & Schuster, 2002.

Huxley, Aldous. *Brave New World and Brave New World Revisited*. Reissued ed. Combined ed. New York, NY: HarperCollins, 2004.

Mundy, Liza. *Everything Conceivable: How Assisted Reproduction Is Changing Our World*. New York, NY: Knopf, 2007.

Orenstein, Peggy. *Waiting for Daisy: A Tale of 2 Continents, 3 Religions, 5 Infertility Doctors, an Oscar, an Atomic Bomb, a Romantic Night, and One Woman's Quest to Become a Mother*. New York, NY: Bloomsbury USA, 2007.

Orr, Tamra. *Science on the Edge—Test Tube Babies*. Farmington Hills, MI: Blackbirch Press, 2003.

Picoult, Jodi. *My Sister's Keeper*. New York, NY: Atria, 2004.

Stone, Katherine. *Carolyn's Journal*. Waterville, ME: Thorndike Press, 2006.

Winkler, Kathleen. *High-Tech Babies: The Debate Over Assisted Reproductive Technology*. Berkeley Heights, NJ: Enslow Publishers, Inc., 2006.

Zack, Kim. *Reproductive Technology*. Farmington Hills, MI: Lucent Books, 2004.

BIBLIOGRAPHY

Ahman, Norhayati Haji. "Assisted Reproduction—Islamic Views on the Science of Procreation." *Eubios Journal of Asian and International Bioethics*, 2003. Vol. 13, pp. 59–60.

American Fertility Association. "Beyond Sex Education: Teens Talk About Their Origins." April 2003. Retrieved March 13, 2008 (http://www.afafamilymatter.com/blogs/index. php?blog=2&cat=19).

American Society of Reproductive Medicine. "Patient Fact Sheet: Intracytoplasmic Sperm Injection (ICSI)." 2001. Retrieved February 10, 2008 (http://www.asrm.org/patients/ FactSheets/ICSI-fact.pdf).

American Society of Reproductive Medicine Ethics Committee. "Preconception Gender Selection for Non-Medical Reasons." *Fertility and Sterility*, Vol. 75, No. 5, May 2001, pp. 861–864.

BBC News. "Baby Son Joy for Test-Tube Mother." January 14, 2007. Retrieved February 9, 2008 (http://news.bbc.co.uk/1/ hi/uk/6260171.stm).

Brian. "Son of a Surrogate." Retrieved March 14, 2008 (http:// sonofasurrogate.tripod.com).

Child Birth Solutions, Inc. "Understanding Your Most Fertile Time." Retrieved February 8, 2008 (http://www. childbirthsolutions.com/articles/preconception/ understanding/Index.php).

Gaines, Deborah. "Fertility and Your Age." 2007. Retrieved January 28, 2008 (http://health.discovery.com/centers/ pregnancy/americanbaby/fertilityandage.html).

Goodwin, Jan. "When It Takes More Than Two—Third Party Reproduction and the Law." *Conceive*, Spring 2005. Retrieved January 3, 2008 (http://wwwlreproductivelawyer. com/news/whenittakes.htm).

HealthDay. "Smoking Before, After, Pregnancy Harm's Daughter's Fertility." November 21, 2007. Retrieved December 24, 2007 (http://www.healthday.com/Articles.asp?AID=610279).

Marriage and Family Encyclopedia. "Assisted Reproductive Technologies—Ethical and Religious Perspective of ARTs." Retrieved February 19, 2008 (http://family.jrank.org/pages/113/Assisted-Reproductive-Technologies-Ethical-Religious-Perspectives-on-ARTs.html).

Mayo Clinic. "Infertility." June 29, 2007. Retrieved December 24, 2007 (http://www.mayoclinic.com/infertility/D500310).

Merrick, Janna, and Robert Blank. *Reproductive Issues in America: A Reference Handbook.* Santa Barbara, CA: ABC-Clio, Inc., 2003.

Mundy, Liza. "Souls on Ice." *Mother Jones*, July/August 2006. Retrieved January 3, 2008 (http://www.motherjones.com/news/feature/2006/07/souls_on_ice.html).

Potter, Daniel, and Jennifer Hanin. *What to Do When You Can't Get Pregnant.* New York, NY: Marlow and Company, 2005.

President's Council on Bioethics. "Reproduction and Responsibility: The Regulation of New Biotechnologies." Retrieved February 8, 2008 (http://www.bioethics.gov/reports/reproductionandresponsibility.html).

Reuters Health Information. "Obesity Hurts a Woman's Chances of Conception." December 12, 2007. Retrieved December 24, 2007 (http://www.reuters.com/article/healthnews/idUSN1155920920071212).

ScienceBlog.com. "Multiple Births—Their Risks and How to Prevent Them." July 2002. Retrieved February 16, 2008 (http://www.scienceblog.com/community/older/2002/F/20022305.html).

Shaw, Anita. "Designer Babies: What Do Teens Think?" *Science and Public Affairs*, September 2005. Retrieved March 14, 2008 (http://www.intute.ac.uk/healthandlifesciences/iscicom/BIBNovember_2005.html).

Smietana, Robert. "400K and Counting." *Christianity Today*, Vol. 47, No.7, June 2003, p.17.

Spar, Debora. *The Baby Business*. Boston, MA: Harvard Business School Publishing, 2006.

Stenson, Jacqueline. "Birds and Bees for 'Test Tube' Babies." MSNBC, July 23, 2003. Retrieved March 14, 2008 (http://www.msnbc.msn.com/id/3076785).

Tarkan, Laurie. "Lowering Odds of Multiple Births." *New York Times*, February 19, 2008. Retrieved February 20, 2008 (http://www.nytimes.com/2008/02/19/health/19multiple.html).

U.S. Census Bureau. "Population Statistics." January 28, 2008. Retrieved January 28, 2008 (http://www.census.gov/population/www/popclockus.html).

U.S. News. "Teen Birth Rates Up for First Time in 14 Years, U.S. Reports." December 5, 2007. Retrieved February 3, 2008 (http://health.usnews.com/usnews/health/healthday/071205/teen-birth-rate-up-for-first-time-in-14-years-us-reports.htm).

Van Dusen, Allison. "Men's and Women's Fertility Facts— Explained." *Forbes*, April 11, 2007. Retrieved January 15, 2008 (http://www.forbes.com/2007/04/10/fertility-men-women-forbeslife-cx_avd_0411fertility.html).

Wahrman, Miryam. "Assisted Reproduction and Judaism." Jewish Virtual Library, 2008. Retrieved February 19, 2008 (http://www.jewishvirtuallibrary.org/jsource/Judaism/ivf.html).

Walter, James, and Thomas Shannon. *Contemporary Issues in Bioethics: A Catholic Perspective*. Lanham, MD: Rowen and Littlefield, 2005.

World Health Organization. *WHO Laboratory Manual for the Examination of Human Semen and Sperm-Cervical Mucus Interaction*. 4th ed. Cambridge, England: Cambridge University Press, 1999.

INDEX

A

adoption, 6, 12, 43, 48
  of embryos, 6, 46, 47–48
age, and effect on fertility, 13, 14, 28
American Fertility Association, 34, 45
American Society for Reproductive
    Medicine, 31, 32, 40
assisted reproductive technology
    (ART), 28–34
  cost of, 42, 43
  moral and ethical concerns about,
    35–41, 43, 45, 47
  who it is recommended for, 28–29

B

Bernstein, Anne, 34
birth statistics, 4
body mass index, 17
  calculating, 16
Brown, Leslie and John, 29–31
Brown, Louise Joy, 30, 31

C

Centers for Disease Control and
    Prevention, 4
chlamydia, 19
conception, and timing, 9–10, 12, 24

D

"designer" babies, 6, 40–41, 50

E

eating disorders, 21

ectopic pregnancy, 14, 19
Edwards, Robert, 29, 31
embryo adoption, 6
embryos
  adoption of, 6, 46, 47–48
  formation of, 11
  freezing of, 31, 43, 46–47, 49, 50
endometriosis, 20
estrogen, 10

F

fallopian tubes, 7–8, 24
  blockage of and infertility, 19–20,
    23, 28
female reproductive anatomy, 7–9
Fisch, Dr. Harry, 14
follicle stimulating hormone (FSH),
    10, 25

G

Gaines, Deborah, 14
gender selection, 37–40, 41, 50

H

Hanin, Jennifer, 22
hormones, 10–11, 25
  imbalance of, 20–21

I

infertility
  causes of, 13–21
  definition of, 5
  female, 13, 14, 17, 19–21

About the Author

Dr. Linda Bickerstaff, a University of Missouri–trained general surgeon, has cared for women with salpingitis, tubal pregnancies, endometriosis, and polycystic ovarian syndrome. Writing this book increased her awareness of how devastating these problems can potentially be to those who want to have children.

Photo Credits

Cover Schering AG/Getty Images; cover (inset) © www. istockphoto.com/dra_schwartz; pp. 5, 15 © Shutterstock.com; p. 8 © L. Birmingham/Custom Medical Stock Photo; p. 10 Yorgos Nikas/Stone/Getty Images; p. 11 Nucleus Medical Art, Inc./Getty Images; p. 18 Anderson Ross/Digital Vision/Getty Images; p. 19 © Hans-Ulrich Osterwalder/Photo Researchers, Inc.; p. 20 © www.istockphoto.com/Ken Hurst; p. 23 © Alix/ Photo Researchers, Inc.; p. 26 © Dr. Najeeb Layyous/Photo Researchers, Inc.; p. 29 Saeed Khan/AFP/Getty Images; p. 30 Keystone/Getty Images; p. 32 Per-Anders/Getty Images; pp. 36, 41, 44, 48 © AP Images; p. 39 Keith Weller/USDA; p. 47 Robyn Beck/AFP/Getty Images; p. 49 David McNew/Getty Images.

Designer: Evelyn Horovicz; Cover Designer: Nelson Sá;
Editor: Kathy Kuhtz Campbell; Photo Researcher: Amy Feinberg